Ashley Fitzgerald

YOGA:

THE BASICS

A beginner's guide to lose weight, relief stress, prevent disease, increase metabolism and find your peace within using the millenary exercises that have endured the test of time."

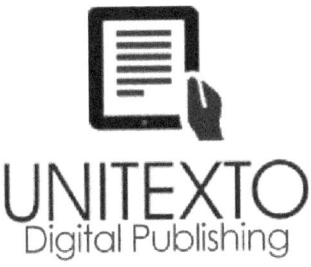

UNITEXTO
Digital Publishing

TABLE OF CONTENTS

I0428388

Introduction

Yoga is the ancient mind-body practice thought to have originated in the East. It has become increasingly popular here in the West, and has developed into a lasting favorite for many people. It's no wonder.

With Yoga, the body is strengthened and toned, greater perseverance is achieved as well as a sense of peace and serenity of mind. The mental facilities are sharpened, as greater oxygen flow increases the health and food supply becomes available to all of the cells of the body. Coupled with meditation, Yoga is a force for calmness of mind, and the foundation for an active and fit body.

Many people have gotten into shape with the help of Yoga. It can spark a lifelong dedication to health and wellness and increase awareness for all of the actions one undertakes in life, including those that may be harmful, which in turn leads to the ability to rectify any harmful behaviors. Knowledge is power, including the power to take control of one's own life and health. The habit of overeating and eating unhealthy items requires awareness to tackle it, and Yoga can bring about this awareness.

 Also, once you start out with one track of fitness, you often become inspired to try other forms of exercise. This could take the form of dancing, running, mountain climbing, skiing, etc. Many people who struggled with extreme obesity have been able to incorporate high-intensity sports into their lives, sports they never dreamed they could do. Yoga is low impact and, as such, a good way to begin an exercise program if you've never done much off of the couch before.

Yoga can help with a lot of things, but what you need is a personal commitment to change and to maintaining that change. If you put your time and effort into a Yoga practice and consistently stick to a healthy diet, you can expect fast results.

Chapter One: What is Yoga?

A perception some people have before really finding out about Yoga, is people twisting themselves into pretzels, contortionists performing acrobatic and impressive feats. Sure, you get to stretch out quite a bit with Yoga. It's true that you push your physical limits in a lot of ways. However, it's not for looks, not for show and definitely not for impressing anyone and competing with anyone (not even yourself). It's about bettering yourself, developing yourself to your full potential and awakening your awareness. You go through life with a clear mind, a balanced body and with a better sense of your feelings. Yoga helps to connect these elements of the self to facilitate health and a sense of awareness.

There are many different types of Yoga. What most people in the western world think of as Yoga, is usually Hatha Yoga, which consists of doing a routine of poses accompanied by inhalation and exhalation connected with each pose. Other types of Yoga that involve movement and breathing include Kundalini Yoga which consists of repetitive motions.

Mind, body, spirit development

Physical Yoga (or Asanas) is what we normally call Yoga. These poses and body movements connected with the breath build strength and bring oxygen to the cells, muscles and organs of the body. But there are other aspects of the yogic path which are even more fundamental.

Traditionally, there were two steps before the Asanas to observe before the student was allowed to proceed to the physical exercises. Number one is Yama. This is how one deals with other people. It means "universal morality".

Number two is Niyama, and this is how one deals with the self. It is required in the teachings of Yoga to treat the self and others with kindness. Once this foundation was attained, then the student could begin a physical practice of Yoga consisting of the exercises most people associate with Yoga.

In the West, we usually start out exercising the body and then learn about the other aspects and hopefully apply them, since they are very helpful in balancing the mind and spirit, finding peace in the self and being committed to peace in the world. It's OK to start out with the physical aspect and move on to the others afterward.

The next step in the eight limbed path of Yoga is Pranayama, and this is also often learnt in the context of a typical Yoga class. Pranayama is the control of the breath, which is linked to the universal life force, also called Prana. (The Chinese refer to Prana as Chi or Qi). Pratyahara is the control of the senses, Dharana is the turning inward of the senses, Dhyana is meditation concentrated on the divine, and lastly, Samadhi is the uniting with the divine. What we will discuss the most in this book are Asanas and Pranayama, but we'll also touch upon the preceding limbs of Yoga, namely Yama and Niyama.

Self care
When we get started doing Yoga, we naturally begin to pay attention to the body. We notice where we are tense, what muscles are tight, where it might be difficult to breathe.

Maybe we turned to Yoga after an injury or a traumatic stage of life. In this case, we already naturally begin to tune into ourselves in a different way. This is a natural, intuitive observing of Niyami, the observance of the self. We breathe, and allow ourselves to just be. We see where we are at any given moment, and come to accept that. By accepting that, we can move onto other things; we are no longer attached. We come into the present moment and can move to the next moment with grace.

Some of the specific ways we can take better care of ourselves in relation to Yoga also occur off the mat.

Physical strength

Letting go of mental clutter and overcoming laziness and other barriers that are of the mind allow us to build on our actual physical strength. We get the mental power to build on our physical power so we can move through life feeling better.

Mental well-being

The deep breathing that comes with a proper Yoga practice helps the mind to relax, and enables peace to take over.

A sense of the spirit

Yogis and Yoginis (a Yogini is a female practitioner of Yoga) often start out just doing physical exercise to get in shape, but find a sense of spirituality after developing a commitment to the practice. They start to see life in a new way, and get inspired by various spiritual teachings out there.

While it is no guarantee that you will become interested in this aspect, many people become ignited by the world of Yoga and find a new angle on life.

Chapter Two: A Spiritual Legacy of Health

A History

Yoga has been practiced for thousands of years. It may be even older than we think. The first mention of Yoga in the oldest text in the world: the Rig-Veda. Some images from Shamanism depict Yoga as well, and Yoga has roots in Hinduism and Buddhism. As such, mankind has been reaping the benefits of Yoga for a very long time.

Types of Yoga

There are many types of Yoga, with some being relatively traditional and others being somewhat modern. They all have their roots in the ancient teachings and their principles date back to the start.

Hatha Yoga combines the Pranayama breathing exercises with a set of poses (Asanas) to prepare the mind and body for meditation and is generally gentle and good for beginners.

Vinyasa Yoga is yoga with synchronized breathing so that each movement corresponds to either an inhalation or exhalation. It is great for getting energy moving.

Ashtanga Yoga also contains synchronized breathing with Asanas, but consists of series of poses that are consistent. For example, one series may contain 7 poses performed in succession and will always be the same in that series. The primary series is for beginners, and further series become

11

more challenging. It is rigorous and energizing, great if you want to train to do more challenging sports like running and need to first acquire stamina.

Kundalini Yoga is a dynamic form of Yoga, consisting of repeated movements called Kriyas. This type of Yoga combines mantra chanting, meditation and dynamic breathing techniques with the Kriyas. The Kriya exercises are synchronized with the breath and are designed to awaken the energy in the spine, which is thought to lead to increased awareness and health.

Iyengar Yoga focuses on the details of each pose or Asana in order to get the optimal alignment for each one. A number of props (blocks, blankets, belts, chairs) can be used in order to obtain the correct alignment, depending on the person doing the exercises.

Asanas are held for a long time to get the most out of each one, for the benefit of connective tissue, ligaments and muscles that are concerned in each pose.

Yin Yoga also holds each individual pose for a long time, but this form of Yoga takes it to the extreme with each pose being held for five minutes. This helps to stimulate circulation and flexibility and is often very challenging.

Restorative Yoga is a great type of Yoga to do to relax and stretch. If you are in need for a release and a relaxation session, this is the Yoga form for you.

Each pose is easy to do, and designed to totally let go of any tension.

Poses are held for ten minutes, but in a way that feels great and is without strain.

Chapter Three: Yogi Lifestyle (Diet, Practice, Way of Thinking)

To get started with Yoga, find course offerings nearby your hometown or where you are located most of the time. You will want to invest in a Yoga mat and appropriate clothes as well as some props such as a band and blocks. Shoes are not necessary for Yoga as Yoga is performed barefoot. You will want to take water with you to class, but it is said that drinking during a Yoga session changes the flow of energy. At any case, if you feel super thirsty you will want to take a sip. You might try drinking a lot before and after class.

What do yogis and yoginis eat?

Yogis and Yoginis eat a healthy diet rich in fruit and vegetables, organic where possible, and drink lots of water and avoid harmful substances such as alcohol and drugs. Traditionally, a yogic diet is vegetarian. For some people it may be difficult or unreasonable to totally give up meat from one day to the next, so a step in the right direction would be to go without meat 1-2 days a week and perhaps increase from there. Sugar and caffeine are substances some Yogis and Yoginis go without, while others enjoy their green tea from time to time. Again, it's a matter of taking it slowly and first looking at health from a holistic standpoint, and doing what's right for you and your health while taking other beings into consideration.

A good yogic breakfast might be:

An organic fruit smoothie or organic homemade oatmeal with apple slices

Lunch:

A salad with goat cheese and plenty of green vegetables

Dinner:

A spicy lentil soup with a veggie wrap

How often to practice Yoga?

Generally, the more often and the longer you practice Yoga the better. You will want to see how you feel after every session, and also during each pose. Make sure you breathe deeply and fully. If you are in any pain or fear injury, stop. Also, when starting out, it's important to consult a doctor if you have any injuries or potential problems. You will also want to start by attending a class so a teacher can check your alignment to prevent injury. This is crucial. Once you have attended some classes and have gotten a feel for the alignment, you can start your home practice and make it a regular part of your routine. Any lifestyle change requires dedication to doing it correctly, to make sure the effects are positive and healing.

Where to do Yoga?

Start out by researching places in your hometown that offer Yoga classes. Your local fitness studio might be one option. Once you have taken some Yoga classes with a professional teacher, you can start doing Yoga anywhere and you can develop your home practice to address the parts of your body that are stiff or less flexible.

Home practice

To start out with Yoga at home and in class at a Yoga studio, you will need to invest in a Yoga mat. You can find inexpensive ones online and in many department stores. They come in a variety of colors or designs, so you can find something that speaks to your personal style. Clothes should be comfortable but not too loose. You can find clothes specifically designed for doing Yoga at a wide array of stores and online shops.

To get your home practice started, you can select a Yoga flow from class and expand on it, look at videos online, or take some of the poses explained in this book.

Chapter Four: Sun salutations to start the day

Once you've started taking classes in person and have consulted a Yoga instructor, you can introduce Yoga into your daily workout routine. The best way to start your day, wake up all of your muscles, increase awareness for the day and oxygenate your blood is to do the sun salutations routine (also known as Surya Namaskar in Sanskrit, the language of ancient Hinduism and Yoga).

You can just roll out of bed, roll out your Yoga mat, breathe deeply, get centered and do this set of Asanas, letting your breath lead you in and out of each pose.

1. Mountain
   Perform the mountain pose by standing up straight. Spread your toes, firm your legs, move your shoulders up, back and down so your chest is lifted. Your feet are either together, or just at shoulder width, slightly apart. Bring your hands to prayer pose (palms together at the level of the heart). Breathe in and out with your eyes closed. Open them and proceed to the next Asana.
2. Extend in Mountain
   As you inhale deeply, move your arms up, raised over your head, bending your back slightly backward. Your palms face each other.
3. Swan dive to bend forward

17

From the extended mountain position, exhale and bring your upper body forward. If you are more flexible, try to bring your nose to your knees. If you are tight in the knees, go ahead and bend them slightly. (Don't force this pose since doing it wrong or doing it with too much force can cause back trouble.) As you bend, bring your arms by your sides and bend from the waist. If you can, touch the floor and if you are feeling too tight in the knees go ahead and rest your hands on your ankles.

4. Inhale and look forward with your head.

5. Exhale and return to the forward bend position from number 3.

6. Plank pose

   Move into a push-up like position while inhaling. Stay in the up position. The shoulders are over the wrists, the abs are in, the feet flexed and the toes spread.

7. Lower yourself to the ground while exhaling, but keep your chest and knees raised. The elbows are kept in, close to the ribcage.

8. Cobra pose

   Inhale with the lower body now lowered to the ground (lower body resting on the ground) and raise the upper body (the pose resembles a cobra). The chest is lifted, the elbows are still close to the ribs. The thighs are firm, the knee caps activated. The shoulders are rolled back, the shoulder blades down.

9. Downward facing dog

Exhale and move into downward facing dog. The palms are pressed into the Yoga mat, and the fingers are spread (activating the muscles). The hands are under the shoulders. Lift the hips and straighten the legs slowly and gently with the heels pressing into the mat. The body forms an inverted V. Remain in this pose for a few breaths.

10. Inhale and step forward so that you are in the forward bend Asana once more. Look forward.
11. Exhale and relax in forward bend.
12. Inhale and roll up from the waist, with the arms moving synchronized to the breath so that they finish above the head so you are in the extended mountain pose.
13. Exhale and bring down the arms so they finish in prayer pose, with the palms together in front of the heart.
14. Repeat these Asanas several times, taking care to breathe deeply. Move decisively, but gently, firmly yet with care.

Yoga is about balancing energy with calmness and peace, firmness with gentleness. The practitioner finds balance of the body, and balance of the feelings and the thoughts. Part of the reason for this is the steady breath maintained throughout is relaxing and counters tension. If you have stress (as most people do in this fast-paced modern world) then you can benefit from a regular Yoga practice.

Specific exercises to relieve pain

One of the great things about Yoga is that you can perform exercises to prevent and heal health problems including physical pain. Here are some of the best exercises for targeting specific problems.

Yoga poses for migraines and headaches:

Standing forward fold:

Like the standing forward bend, you inhale and raise your arms above your head. Exhale and bend from the waist. Let your spine relax and your head hang down. Bend your knees if you need to. Grab the opposite elbow with your right hand, the right elbow with the left hand. Let everything just hang down and breathe deeply. You will find you go deeper into the pose automatically. Stay in the pose as long as it feels good. This helps loosen tension that causes headaches and migraines.

Child's pose

Here's another great restorative pose that eases tension and helps you relax (which in turn mitigates stress and tension-related headaches and migraines.) It's easy and simple for beginner's. Kneel down with the knees just slightly apart. Put the arms in front of you and stretch them out long and let your head rest on the ground. Breathe deeply and stay here as long as you like, at least for give breaths.

Legs Against the Wall

Sit down next to a wall and move onto your side. Gently roll over so you are on your back with legs resting against the wall. Let your arms stretch out to the sides and breathe deeply.

Exercises to stimulate weight loss
Bridge Pose

Lie on the back with the arms stretched out at the sides. Bring the knees up with the feet still flat on the floor. Raise the buttocks off the floor (the arms are still at the sides). Lift so that your stomach and chest are also elevated. Inhale while raising the body upward. Breathe out and in a few times while holding the pose. Repeat 10 times to activate the metabolism.

Boat pose

This is one of the best exercises you can do to strengthen the abs. Sit down with the legs stretched out in front of you. Bring the legs together, then lift them off of the floor. You can use your hands to support this motion. The body forms a v with the formation of the upper body and legs. Take your hands off of the floor if you can and hold the pose. Breathe deeply in and out and hold for at least five breaths.

Cobra pose

Lay on the stomach and place the hands next to the sides (close to the ribs). Inhale and lift the upper body using the stomach muscles. The shoulders are up and back. The head is the last thing to come up. The palms are under the shoulders, the thigh muscles activated, the feet flexed or pointed out behind you.

Seated forward bend

Sit down with your legs stretched out in front of you. Inhale, raise your arms above your head. Exhale and bend forward, grabbing your toes if you are able. Go gently and don't overextend. Let your head touch your knees.

Poses for a good night's sleep

Child's Pose

Child's pose is great because it allows the body to relax completely. Deep breaths help the mind to relax. Kneel on the floor, allow your head to rest on the floor and stretch the arms out straight in front of you. Let all stress and tension simply wash away with the deep breath.

Raised Leg

A pose you can do from the Yoga mat, and even in bed, is the Raised Leg. You will want to use a scarf or a Yoga band to perform this. Lay down on your back and raise one leg up at a 90 degree angle. Wrap the band or scarf around your foot and hold it with both hands, pulling the band toward you. Allow your foot and leg muscles to counteract the force. Repeat on the other side.

Wide-Legged Standing Forward Bend

From mountain pose (standing straight with the shoulders back), spread the legs wide (about 4 feet apart or five if you are a taller person). Exhale and bend forward from the hips. Spread the arms also wide so that you are touching the floor almost in line with the feet. Your fingertips should be touching the floor and the elbows bent. Rest your head on a Yoga block (this can be ordered online or purchased in sporting goods shops). Stay here for a few breaths, then come up by rooting down into the feet and rising up slowly.

Yoga to Fight Anxiety
Bound Angle Pose

This pose is also great for loosening up tight hips and counteracting the effects of sitting in a chair all day.

Start by sitting on your Yoga mat with your legs out in front of you. (You can sit on a towel or other item to elevate the hips if you feel unusually tight there). Move the feet toward you and drop the knees outward while bringing the feet together. Your hands hold the toes. Breathe deeply in and out. To go deeper into this pose, bend forward slightly.

Yoga to Improve Digestion
Head to Knee Forward Bend

Sit on your Yoga mat with your legs stretched out in front of you. Inhale and bright the right sole of the foot in against the left thigh, just above the knee. Exhale. Now inhale and raise your arms above your head. Exhale and bend forward. Stay here for a few breaths. Then switch and repeat on the other side.

Poses for a positive mood and outlook
Warrior I pose

Stand with the legs apart. The right foot is pivoted to point outward, the left foot faces forward. Inhale and raise the arms overhead, bend the right knee so that it is over the right ankle like a lunge. (Now you are facing in the direction your right foot is pointing, with the upper body.) Stay in this position inhaling and exhaling. Then repeat on the other side.

Chapter Five: Why Meditation is a Part of Yoga

Yoga may seem like pure physical exercise, but what it does for the mind is an extremely important component. In fact, in Eastern philosophy, the spirit and the mind would be the more important aspects whereas the physical aspect is just the icing on the cake. In the West it tends to be the opposite, but we don't need to feel bad about that. However, we should take care to build in meditation to our Yoga practice so we can reap the full rewards Yoga can provide to living a balanced life.

What is meditation?

Meditation is a state of calm of the mind where thoughts either stop or slow down. Meditation allows worries to fade, for fears to clear and for silence to come in.

Modern research has confirmed many of the numerous benefits meditation provides. It has shown that meditation enhances memory and reduces or eliminates stress. In addition, many believe that meditation leads to increased awareness and a kindling of spirituality. It is thought to balance the brain. Without a doubt, it facilitates relaxation. A relaxed life is a more happy life.

How to meditate

Meditation can be done seated or lying down. Some people find it difficult to relax completely when sitting down, and

25

others find it hard to stay awake and wind up falling asleep when lying down. Find the position that suits you best. You will want to relax totally, and be completely laidback in the body but still totally aware in the mind. Your thoughts will slow, but you will remain conscious, simply observing your breath.

To start, take a seat or lay down in a comfortable position. Breathe deeply, in and out. Repeat that and begin to observe your breath simply coming and going.

A guided meditation

Take a seat or lay down. Inhale fully, exhale completely. Let all tension and stress simply leave the body. Concentrate first on the toes and imagine all tension leaving them. Then imagine tension slipping away from the rest of your foot, part by part. Then move up to the ankles. Visualize and feel tension leaving each part of your body, ending with the head. Now notice your breath. It rises and falls like the waves of the ocean. Hear the waves washing onto the shore. The silver moon shines above you. Now imagine you are enveloped by the silver light of the moon. The silver light cleanses and refreshes you and lends you serenity. Feel comforted and secure. Simply enjoy the peace this brings you.

Quiet time for the mind

Our daily lives are so fast-paced these days. We rush to work, we rush to meetings and we hurry through our meals. We rarely have the time to simply BE. We have to schedule time to be with our family members. It's a hard era to live in. Yoga helps us to manage stress, to find a time to simply be in the moment. Meditation compliments and completes the process of finding inner calm and coming to the present moment.

Benefits of meditation

Meditation is an essential part of the Eastern religions. Buddhists and Hindus meditate daily, sometimes several times a day. It would be unheard of to perform Yoga without meditation. As Yoga strengthens the body and helps to detox, so does meditation do for the mind. This way we can balance ourselves totally and come to our full potential; body, mind and spirit.

Chapter Six: Mantra

The mantra is an essential part of Kundalini Yoga. But it can be done in the context of any type of Yoga. You can start your Yoga practice, or close your practice with a mantra and then proceed with meditation. You can speak a mantra or sing a mantra. It helps to calm the brain waves and the vibrations of singing in the head help clear the sinuses. It has many physical and mental benefits.

You can find a variety of "traditional" mantras out there. One is " Sat Nam" which simply means I am. This helps you to connect to the present moment. Another powerful mantra that has withstood the test of time is the famous "Om". Most people are familiar with this mantra, and with good reason. It brings us in tune with the resonance of the universe. (This has even been tested, so this is science). Om resonates at 432 Hertz, the pitch of the universe. This tunes the mind and brings us in greater harmony with the world around us.

You can also make up your own mantra in English, or whatever language feels best or is best suited to your purposes. You might make up a mantra such as "I am peace" or "I am beautiful", "I am worthy and loved", etc. You want your Yoga practice to give you strength and energy, so find a mantra that will build you up positively. This way you can face your life with radiance and a great attitude.

Some say mantra is "medicine for the soul". This way, you have meditation for the mind, a physical Yoga practice for the body, and also have something for the soul. You can affect your being positively on several fronts with a comprehensive Yoga practice.

Chapter Seven: Further Benefits and Inspiration

Yoga has so many positive effects on the life of the practitioner. You don't have to do extremely advanced poses to get the full benefits out of a Yoga practice. Some people find that when they start Yoga, they start getting interested in other forms of physical sports. They start running or skiing or even playing tennis. Couch potatoes can use Yoga to get going and from there built up to other things, since it is mild and gentle on knees and other joints.

Since Yoga is not only physical, but mental and spiritual, some people also find a renewed interest in the religion they grew up with, or find a new form of spirituality. Yoga opens doors and windows and brings new perspectives on life.

How to keep motivated?

There are lots of things you can do to keep your interest in Yoga going. You can attend classes with friends, or try new classes and styles of Yoga. You can find videos online to do, and read books on Yoga. You can change up your practice, and maybe try doing it in a heated room to make it more strenuous if you need a challenge. If you feel like your practice is too strenuous, try some restorative poses. You can also post to online groups and get moral support from others with an interest in Yoga.

What Yoga will do for you over the long run?

Yoga will make your body more flexible, and stronger too. You will breathe more deeply and have more awareness. You might notice more the way your food tastes, and take a greater interest in your health than ever before. You might become really interested in Yoga and try several different styles. If you stick with your practice, you will discover a lot of positive results that you might never have expected and your life path changed in a good way.

Where you can do Yoga and find Yoga?

You can find Yoga everywhere these days! You can do Yoga from online videos in your own living room. Some cities offer free Yoga in the park where a lot of people meet up and do Yoga together outdoors. Exercising outside is particularly beneficial since you have increase oxygen and the added bonus of vitamin D from the sun. There are Yoga studios in every town, and almost everyone knows someone who already does Yoga. You can talk to your friends and get valuable tips on where to go to get started, or how to continue your practice if you are looking for a new challenge or something exciting and new to try.

Conclusion

Yoga is like a sport, but is so much more than that. It isn't about competition, it isn't about showing off. It is about realizing your own personal potential and finding greater comfort, strength and awareness that comes completely from within. Of course, you can use tools that come from the outside (such as from books such as this one) or find inspiration from other people (like Yoga instructors, friends and family). The ultimate spark and will to continue on any path has to come from within, and it is finding that strength that comes from within that Yoga is all about. Balance is another element that Yoga instills in us, and we find this by balancing strength with flexibility. We are strong and flexible like a tree that bends in the wind but does not break.